The YOU After... BABY

The YOU After...BABY
Copyright © 2018 by Sally Donovan

No part of this publication may be reproduced, distributed, or transmitted in any form or by any means, including photocopying, recording, or other electronic or mechanical methods, without the prior written permission of the author, except in the case of brief quotations embodied in critical reviews and certain other non-commercial uses permitted by copyright law.

ISBN: 978-1-77532-910-7 (Paperback)

The YOU After...BABY

A sacred "*scribery*" for the sassy new Mamma.

The Mom journal—a guidance counsellor for adjusting to the new YOU, post-procreation. While the emphasis on all you gain in life as a Mother is rightfully unyielding, let's acknowledge that after having a child you may feel you have lost part of your identity.

As you step into motherhood there may be days you miss parts of the old YOU. Well here is your no-judgement zone to help you deal with that and all the very natural and, yes, varying states of mind that you will find yourself in along the way. With time, some applications and perspective, like stretch marks, uncertainties will fade. Let this be one tool to help you with that, to manage all those feelings with some insight for your mind, and a few jabs for your funny bone.

Use your emotions to format your journal, and be inspired by some of my personal experiences, a few conventional insights, and, cynical blurbs too. This is where you write, jot, draw your way to a redefined you.

As you transform your life from the more self-involved, free-to-be woman that is no longer, guess who will be left standing? YOU, as a fantastic MOM.

The new, stronger, better-than-ever YOU!

This journal belongs to:

_____

A MOM as at:

_____

YOU:

FOREVER MORE

From ME to YOU

Here's the thing. I'm a numbers gal and a wee bit social media adverse too. So why am I sharing words and personal stories with you? Why should you use or share this journal, read my quips, use it as a resource for self-expression, or as a tool to help find "YOU" again?

Because above all, I am empathetic, I am passionate, and wholeheartedly believe in THE POWER OF PERSPECTIVE.

I feel compelled to convey personal insights from my "been there, done that" experiences. I feel compelled to help and apply the theory of strength in numbers; you are not alone. Okay, so I tend to be wordy and generally live for a laugh, and this was an ideal platform for that too!

Frankly, it can just suck when you are thrown a life lemon (pardon the pun); or you are in the thick of a major life transition — bad or even good. During these times of change you may feel a loss, whether it's literally part of your life, or parts of your identity. In dealing with that loss, I feel some women may find it difficult to process their thoughts and emotions without judgment, or finding that other "G" spot... yeah, the guilt complex.

During major life transitions of my own, I realized the constructive power of support and validation from others, in all its various forms. Generally, I think we not only crave this backing (secretly or not), but can use it to endure the not-so-certain times in life. I am also a big believer of expression through words, and, yes, often way too many of them!

So it was then that I became passionate about combining these concepts. I wanted to promote the simple keys of comfort that I used while navigating my bumps in the road; to read, write, and, above all, laugh. I wanted to create a support tool and an outlet to rationalize, scream, cry, and revel about life.

My story leading up to this point is a classic tale. I have always been an achiever and goal-oriented individual. Upon graduating university and getting a job, I married my school sweetheart. My career took off and I was climbing a quick ladder to success. But after our first child was born I slowed things down and opted to work part-time, to ensure I could be a fully engaged Mom too; the most prominent, challenging and wonderful role of my life.

My husband's company and career blossomed, we had another child, and I was balancing work and home life with two kids the best I could. We spent years renovating our entire home in a great neighbourhood. We escaped the city and enjoyed his family cottage, travelled, and were part of a huge family and friend network. Life was good, typical, planned, and from anyone who knew us, we were "that" couple.

Then one day it happened. My marriage came to an end. When my world blew up, so to speak, marriage breakdown, followed by my corporate division closing down, I decided the world was trying to tell me something. I took the time to revisit who I was, and, more importantly, who I wanted to be.

I am into the groove of my new normal, from explaining the unexplainable to my kids to taking on life now as a single gal. The roller coaster and path I took to get here today was not easy. My friends and family, an unscathed sense of humour, and the power of perspective guided me on that ride; in fact, all of it made me a better person in the end. That should be the goal of any life transition, a *better YOU...after.*

Now I find myself here on a new journey, to provide support and smiles to those who find themselves in a funk; specifically, women dealing with major life changes I can relate to. I want to hug every single one of them, crack an inappropriate joke, to crack an oh-so-necessary smile. But to do this one person at a time is not convenient as a single mom!

I have heard the words "you should write a book or share your thoughts" more than once in my life.

So this is me, just wanting to spread some optimism wrapped in cynicism to you.

This is your hug.

The YOU After... BABY

"The You After..." journal
by Sally Donovan

So here you are, a Mom.

Congratulations and big hugs to your little one! Welcome to the Mom club; may you wear your newly adorned "tattoo" of Mom-ship with pride. Wish that tattoo wasn't in the form of stretch marks, scars, or stretched parts, but with all good things...

Unlike other journals you may keep to capture each milestone, breath, burp, and bowel movement your baby achieves, per hour, this journal is for YOU.

There will be many emotions that accompany this new Mom role of yours; and in with the NEW means, well, out with some of the OLD. It is hard to expect you can immediately disregard the former YOU after the final "push" to becoming a parent. With the upmost respect and encouragement to new Moms everywhere, I think it is okay to admit that, and more than okay to deal with it head on.

With all the good of being a Mamma (and it is boundless), there may be times you will be in a state of flux over the new state of your nation.

Your sacred "scribery" is set up to help you handle that emotional roller coaster of adjusting to the new YOU. You will experience different feelings at different times, and in no particular direction. That's right, emotions are not logical (sigh, that hurts the left side of my brain).

How and when to scribe your thoughts? Well that is up to you and your new personal time ruler, your baby. You will have to prioritize the emotional benefits of reading and journaling even mere minutes here and there, as you take on this major life transition.

Some moments you will find yourself in will be *confusion, resentment, sadness, and acceptance*. Now let me introduce you to these emotions, my good pals, and who you will meet along your journey to redefining YOU.

OH MY: Confused Cathy.

She is so sweet, you know with that slapped look of shock on her face.

She deals with the surprises and expectations that read as "fake news."

UGH: Jelly Jill.

She is reckless (as in the Jill that pushes others down that damn hill).

She is fuelled by sleep deprivation and her perceptions, rational or not.

BLAH: Betty Blue.

She comes in AND out like a lion OR a lamb — how do you tame that?

She unleashes a fury of sensitivity when you sometimes least expect it.

OH YEAH: The YOU After BABY.

She is in you, just wait and see.

Grateful, confident, changed, and better than ever. Hello, YOU!

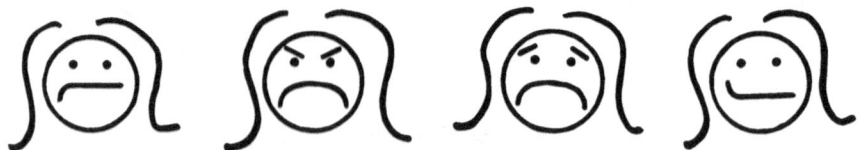

There you go, your new posse.

So whatever MOMENT you are in, take pen to paper to get out your thoughts and clear your mind. Scribe away to help sort through the new YOU.

But above all else, hang on to your sense of humour.

IT WILL SAVE YOUR SOUL!

What Moment Are YOU In?

Oh MY	|	1
Ugh	|	41
Blah	|	79
Oh Yeah	|	117
Hello, YOU!	|	155

In the Moment of...

Oh my

Theory does not always translate to reality.

So, where is the step-by-step e-guide to handle that?

It starts in your closet after you give birth; dismay. Every non-stretchy garment is like a stab to your ego.

For me it actually started in my overnight hospital bag. My favourite PJs were packed for my stay. I was clearly going to slip those pants on right after they pulled (and that they did) my baby out of me. For most of you new Moms out there, I don't need to finish this story. For those who don't know what I am talking about, well count your blessings, skip ahead, and know I am thinking of a few, um, "terms of endearment" that describe that lucky, disciplined, or genetically enriched you.

Apparently, your body needs some time to "settle down." I believe this is the medical term. My hopes of packing away my maternity clothes would have to wait just a little while.

As an analyst by nature, I had been preparing for my upcoming role of Mom. I had the 12 recommended books scattered around the house, dealing with what to expect during pregnancy and the baby's first year. I even had Dr. Seuss's greatest hits. But I can honestly say I was in complete denial about how I would physically and emotionally react in the onset of my baby's debut. My expectations had been established perfectly in my mind...

We would get home to my adorned house with some of my family waiting there. We had prepared pink or blue balloons and ribbons to put outside to announce the arrival of our baby (used the pink, always pink). My husband would carry in the baby sound asleep in the car seat. I would prance in the home filled with flowers and care packages. We would put her down in her new cradle and enjoy the welcome home—maybe even the perfect ray of sunshine would seep through the window. Well, that hopeful and magical scene was just ever-so-slightly different than I imagined.

After my husband's fourth trip to the car with belongings (you do NOT need to pack everything on the "recommended" things to bring to hospital list), we made our way home. We had to stop at the pharmacy to pick up supplies to deal with the oh, let's not promote the odds of, episiotomy, and all the other stuff that happens to you after birth. I had a fully stocked baby medicine cabinet three months prior to delivery day, but barely anything for the delivery woman, namely me.

As my husband ran into the shop, a sad song came on the radio, so I irrationally started crying and sobbed the rest of the way. When we arrived at my home filled with care packages but no one else (my family lives out of town and was dealing with my ailing father), my husband bounced in the house with baby, and me not so bouncing, straggled behind. We laid our baby girl down in a beautiful bassinette and we both smiled. I said, "Welcome home, little one, welcome home." Then I looked around the house. Oh there was sunshine, sunshine streaming around the house, where a tornado had apparently hit in the 48 hours of my absence. End scene.

Reality is not always what we imagine; sometimes it is so, so much more, and other times, it's not even close to par. It is hard work to balance hope and be accepting of the real. But keep gratitude in mind as you settle into Mom mode, and most importantly learn from the valuable experiences along the way. Experience is such a beautiful thing.

Here lay the pages to express the confusion you may have as you try to automatically embrace all things Mom. Write out your questions, thoughts, and hopes for any aspect of this new role and to get back what you think you may have lost: freedom, the ability to wear your fave jeans, or to tackle everything on that to-do list. Even if you think your thoughts are irrational, trivial, or naive, here is your place to let it out. Each day as a new Mom brings on new challenges and "Oh My" moments that are unique to YOU, and so is the way you manage it.

Your new to-do list:

☐ *Keep baby alive*
☐ *Take a shower*

*You catch a glimpse from your window and are drawn in.
You press your hands against the glass. You stare longingly outside.
You see women who are just walking—but they seem free;
no bags, no stroller, and with an overpriced coffee cup in hand.*

You used to be one of "them."

*Kid-free women stalking is only acceptable
for the first year after birth.*

Remember when you thought you were busy BEFORE you had kids?

Changing a diaper seems easy—until you discover the difference between "poop" and "up-the-back-kinda poop."

Breastfeeding takes fast food to another level.

The planning diva in you may have created a list of ALL the things you were going to do in your "free" time, on your maternity leave...

Find the list.
Scrunch it up.
Burn it.
It ain't happening.

How can someone so small rule the entire household?

Getting from A to B will take you an average 25 minutes longer, at any given time of day, for random and multiple reasons.

Get over your past punctuality prestige.
You need to embrace lateness and all that it stands for.
Starting now.

How long does it take to become a fully functioning, engaged employee in a new job?

Now take that number and multiply it by zero.

Motherhood is an evolving process—ask for help, cut yourself some slack, and roll with the punches. You will only master the art of dealing with what life throws your way—and there is no time stamp on that.

*You dressed in pants without a tie string, a decent dinner ready,
a quiet baby, and you in a relaxed state of mind.
Pick ONE.
There will be a period where this will rarely ever exist simultaneously*

In the Moment of...

Ugh

The Prickly Pages.

As in, stay out of the way baby daddy and judgey moms, and I won't prick you with the safety pin now holding my pants closed.

I had a beautiful healthy baby, a fantastic new home, and a hardworking husband—life was grand. Clearly there was no reason for me to ever become irrationally angry at this point in my life? Laugh. Out. Loud.

It is called resentment. And most of the time after becoming a new Mom, I believe some unfounded or founded resentment creeps in. It is usually cast toward the owner of the sperm utilized to make, the now most important person in your life. Ironic, isn't it?

Life isn't fair; it is how you deal with that fact that determines your character, who you really are and how you live life. It's what I've been preaching to my girls for a few years now. (Start scribing your wise parent clichés now for the years to come, because every kid needs to hear a few for the mandated teenager eye-rolling quota.)

I think once you become a Mother, the so-called unfairness factor in life seems to be thrown in your face a bit more, actually like an effing fast ball at times.

Let's see, perhaps it has to do with the delivery aftermath on your body, potentially dealing with breastfeeding, lack of sleep, hormonal imbalance, some isolation and mental shifts, like from calculating logistic regression models, to singing ABC one hundred times a day. There is reason that anger or jealousy, logical or not, will rear its ugly head, into your head. Here is your validation and support to say, this Mom gets it. You will have those moments.

I remember the conversation about the gym like it was yesterday. I will preface the story by mentioning that we had no family living nearby, so go-to support was not easily come by for us. My baby daddy(you may feel the urge to use this term of "endearment" now and again)was trying to explain that after working a very long day, he really needed gym time to get some mental and physical release. Taking a step back I understand his point completely. A more than rational request it would seem, but that was a more than irrational moment in our life.

As I picked at the dried spit-up off my shirt I looked at him, trying to understand his point about him being away from the house for just another couple of hours was not a big deal.

Did he not realize that on some days of Momming, by the end of the afternoon I was watching traffic reports and staring out the window for a car that remotely resembled his? I was checking clocks to ensure none of them had stopped. I needed a mental and physical break from MY entire day (which had no real start or stop time by the way).

The balance of gratitude, joy, and overwhelming love with the evil I call resentment at times is a challenge that will continue forever as a parent. Adjusting to it will take its course. So cut yourself some slack and figure out ways to manage those feelings—writing, talking, long walks, and even longer drinks all do wonders to ease the mind.

If my memory serves me correctly, it was about that time that my husband starting waking up at an ungodly early hour to exercise *before* work. It did seem unfair to him, but we all know what they say about life not being fair...

Here lay the pages to help calm you down when you are well, overwhelmed by the magnitude of being a new Mom. So write, draw pictures, or stab randomly at the pages. Think of this as the cooling off zone before you share your thoughts, words or (let's hope not), stabs with anyone else! This is also a great place to keep a list of all your "over and above the call of Mom duty" moments. Document these to use as ammunition against your child when they are older. You will need all the help you can get.

This section is Rated R for coarse language.

It is okay to admit that in the middle of the night, after three hours of non-stop fussing and crying, you have actually looked for the makings of two small horn buds, growing from the top your baby's head.

*Diaper bag, blanket, wallet, toys, the baby....
and at some point you thought carrying a clutch was a pain.*

1   Alarm.

2   Snooze button.

3   Quiet.

1   Baby crying.

2   Baby crying.

3   Baby crying.

(No, they don't come with buttons.)

*Would it not have made sense to give newborn babies
the ability TO talk to express their ailments,
and then teenagers the ability NOT to talk back?*

Clearly, as a tired, insecure, hormonal, frustrated, brand-new Mom, you are ALWAYS welcoming of unsolicited "expert" know-it-all parenting advice. Please do tell.

Hypothesis: Clocks keep faster time after you bear children.

Observation: Thousands of Mothers utter, "Where does the time go?"

Conclusion: Something has to be going on with parental time keep!

*Sometimes based on the actual manufacturing, storing, and delivering of the baby into the world, Moms have the constitutional right to veto, well, **anything at any time**.*

Sorry, Baby Daddies.

Tip of the day:

*"No, dear, my way of dealing with the baby is not the ONLY way. But my effing four weeks of being the primary caregiver 24/7 may just give me some credentials for you to even CONSIDER I have a point," should be your **inside** voice.*

Your partner is trying.

*Asking your baby to explain what the F*** is the matter is normal.
Seeking for answers at the bottom of a wine bottle is, not so much.*

In the Moment of...

Blah

When rationality takes a hiatus and tissues become scarce.

You've heard about the hormones deal after childbirth. Your body is readjusting to the end of manufacturing a human being. So cut it some slack, because with the dramatic drop in hormones, coupled with sleep deprivation, there will be some emotional flux, and a helluva lot of tears.

Unfortunately for me, the birth of my first daughter was during an unprecedented and very difficult time in my life. My father who had been battling myelodysplasia for two years was losing his fight with the disease. He knew it, my family knew it, and I had tried to mentally ignore it for the previous nine months.

Unspoken words amongst my family had been on our minds for the last few weeks before I gave birth. My father was holding on to meet his youngest grandchild. Then we would lose him. He had only so much fight in him. It was all for her, my baby girl. He died six weeks after her birthday.

It was such a bittersweet time in my life. The sadness of being overwhelmed with a new baby, mixed in with my father's illness, was more than consuming. I had NEVER cried so much in my life. I tried to hide it when I could, but waves of sadness would erupt.

It was not how I imagined. This was not how I planned to bring a life into this world, my world. But it was. Little did I know then, more life lemons were in store for me. But I had this experience of managing that ordeal and coming out somewhat unscathed, and with my baby alive and well! That was proof enough. This was but a moment in my life, and I could handle what the future had in store.

While I hope rearing your child is in the best of circumstances, you will likely still feel waves of emotions come over you. Mental health awareness and openness have emerged more boldly and rightly over the last decade or so. With that should come some comfort in expressing your feelings, especially the sad ones. Here is your acknowledgment to know it is okay to feel anxiety and sadness, and to ask for help if needed.

This is a new job, one where theory and perhaps some "aunting" experience gave you a sense of expectation. But by day three, some of those thoughts and re-read words of expert advice have long left the building. Deal with your state of mind so you can deal with your baby. Forgive yourself for irrational bursts.

Time and effort will not only provide emotional balance but also that valuable stabilizer called experience. Your probation period will soon be over and you will know more than you once did, and you will get the hang of this evolving lifetime role. In the interim, cry if you must—your baby is waterproof for a reason.

Here lay the pages to express yourself when you have that whole ugly cry thing going on, and, yes, it does happen over spilled breast milk! When glum emotions overcome you, get that yuck in your head out on paper. Document your feelings, insecurities, and fears to lift you. Articulate that pit in your stomach caused by all the things that you miss about when you were NOT a Mom and things you can't possibly handle AS a Mom...oh, until you don't and do. But until then, this is your place to unleash the sadness so it doesn't weigh you down so much. This is your safe, non-judgemental, supportive, objective space to let it all out.

Avoid markers here—the text will smear when wet.

*You may have to consider your breasts on loan for awhile.
Sadly, the used and far from original version
are non-exchangeable upon return.*

Sleep—who would have thought this free commodity would be so rare?

Ever wonder how your parents managed to keep you alive without certified car seats, safety locks, foam covers, swingy everything, gates, sleep aids, monitors, cameras, etc., etc., etc.?

Seriously.

*Here lie that "Little Black Dress."
A proper memorial of that LBD you once
rocked is more than appropriate.*

May she R.I.P.

Sleep. Feed. Burp. Change. Repeat.
If only your baby could master what men already know.
(hee hee)

*All good Mammas have a breaking point.
Go on, show your baby who can cry louder.*

_____
_____
_____
_____
_____
_____
_____
_____
_____
_____
_____
_____
_____
_____
_____
_____
_____
_____
_____
_____

Some days I want to wear a t-shirt that provides an explanation for my current state of the nation.

"I used to be smart, and then I had kids."

You now live in a world where spit up is the lesser of two evils.

*You will never appreciate the pause feature
on your TV as much as you do now.*

And yes, reality television is a form of emotional therapy.

In the Moment of...

Oh Yeah

You got this, Mamma.

Now snap your fingers in a Z formation!

I was sitting alone in bed holding my baby girl. I ran my hand over her head and gently down her arm, still in awe that she was here, she was mine. Then as I made my way to her tiny hand she grasped onto my finger. I will always remember that moment. It was the simplest of things, her grabbing onto me. I felt a wave of emotion as I smiled and told her Mommy is here for you...forever.

With all the emotions, uncertainty, newness, and major responsibility that come with being a new Mom, there will be moments when life seems to stop. You simply become mindful of your baby and what an absolute privilege being a Mother can be.

You will also start realizing how much you are evolving. You will learn so much more about yourself after you become a Mother; the *ultimate* in character development and, frankly, living what has meant to be your true life.

Acceptance of anything usually comes with introspective work and the magical elixir of TIME. Your body heals, you master the "routine" only to have it change minutes later, and then master dealing with that too. You realize what is important in life, accept the new challenges and embrace glorious moments of pride ahead, sometimes with grace, and sometimes with not so much.

My belief is that for most women, the second that umbilical cord is cut your Mamma Bear instinct kicks in. You are immediately transformed into a new person with super Mom power. Unlike Wonder Woman, there is not a costume that is adorned instantly with the full power that comes with it. It's simply in you when you need it. Believing in that will help you master your new role better than ever. Especially on the days where a costume to hide from the world would be so effing ideal!

Moms also need their super powers and good judgement to navigate this world of excess knowledge too. What seems your only connection to the outside world at times, filled with information to provide forward thinking, can also hinder your growth as an awesome Mom.

Social media can wake up insecurities, slap you with pre-Mom life desires, and bring on a whole level of obscure questions. All based on mere filtered pictures, and cartooned hand gestures and faces. I want to suggest that accepting who you are and need to be for your baby is solely your business. Period.

From that first time you held your baby in your arms until the rest of your life, as unique as you are, so will be your experience as a Mother. Take the time to be in YOUR moment, and simply enjoy it.

Here lay the pages to revel in your new-found confidence in being a Mom. Congratulations, you did it!

Whether it be a few minutes or many weeks of acceptance you can write about, you can still taste the transformation. This is the holding place for your personal positive clichés on steroids. Write about the hurdles you overcame, the overwhelming good of the now, and the excitement of having the privilege to nurture your baby for years to come.

This section is best enjoyed with a fine wine on a particularly good hair day.

The FIRST smiles, finger grabs, and steps are some of the moments that LAST in your heart forever.

Education = Lessons + Exams
Driver's License = Laws + Hands-On Testing
Sport = Rules + Practice
Parenting = INSTINCT + FEAR (and a dash of HOPE)

Pre-Baby Weekends: Late to bed, late to rise.
Post-Baby Weekends: Early to bed, who's kidding who?

Consistent sleep patterns shall be a memory for awhile.

Let's all say it together.
Rearing a baby is WORK.
The fact that you do this at HOME does not trivialize
the magnitude or impact of the ROLE, which is
in fact the very foundation of society.

You don't need a business card to declare any of that.

There has to be a direct connection between the placenta and a woman's limbic system within her brain.

As the placenta is expelled from her body, so goes part of her full functioning and acute memory as she knew it.

*Welcome to the world of unconditional love.
It's a beautiful thing.*

Take pictures to remind yourself of the happy moments that come with this gig. Yeah, your memory sucks after having children.

Document, document, document!

*Repeat after me: wine bottles are not like fortune cookies.
There are no parental words of wisdom waiting inside.*

Shortly after you have your baby, there will be THE moment. There is no pre-determined time, action, or location for it.

The gesture between YOU and your baby will melt your heart, make you feel invincible, beyond resourceful, and shed all doubts.

That moment is when it really hits you, you are now a Mom.

May your captured thoughts serve you well.
Over time you should look back at all of these "moments."

Then you will see how far YOU have evolved,
After BABY!

Hello, YOU!

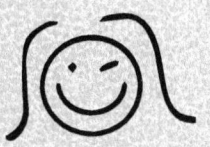

One FINAL Moment

After the birth of both my daughters, I kept a detailed journal about all the firsts of their first year. And, yes, Thing One got much more air time and detail than Thing Two. I am the youngest of four; honestly, I am not sure how my legal documents were even signed off at that time.

I, of course, also kept a journal of my own thoughts through this life change. It was not an easy one as I was dealing with the death of my father too. However, I had witnessed the circle of life and appreciated that my baby was brought into the world when we needed her the most. We called her an angel. She dissipated sadness at times we needed it. A baby can just do that.

In looking through these treasured keepsakes, I noticed that I wrote a letter to my first born, one year after her birth. I remember that is how long it took. It took me a good year to feel like I had found myself again...well my new self with a hip-hugging sidekick. It seems a long time I know, but it can never be a race.

I often remind new Moms that even with all the advice they will hear, this experience is theirs alone. As unique as a baby's fingerprints are the mindsets and circumstances of the parents raising that child.

With some hesitation in sharing my letter, a personal reflection during my passage to Motherhood, I do so in hopes to inspire YOU. Let this be a way to mark this time and your thoughts, of what being a Mom means to you; a way to share inspirations for you and your child, during the inaugural moments of this privileged role.

My Baby Girl,

Thank you. For you have showed me unconditional love, which I felt the day you were born. I will forever be grateful that you changed my heart.

Thank you for being our little angel when we needed you. You brought such light into the world when it felt so dark. You made me a stronger person when I felt like I was grasping for solid ground.

Thank you for making me a new person, a Mom! In an instant you changed my life and priorities. As your Mom I want nothing more than a lifetime of beautiful tomorrows for you. My job is to try and encourage you to be the best person you can be. But I know there will be days when being a good Mom will be hard. So we both need patience, as you mature and make sense of this crazy world.

Of course I wish you a life of good health and happiness, surrounded by people who adore you as much as your parents. But remember to think before you do, be open minded to learn and grow whenever you can, and do so with humility for the awe around us. Believe in yourself, and know your Mom always will.

It will be such a privilege to be a part of your journey as you grow up. But maybe, just maybe for me, you can take your time doing that. Regardless, at one year old to the rest of your life, you will forever be my little angel.

With love and gratitude that you are mine,

Mom

Let this be your space for your thoughts to your baby, and to YOU now, as a new Mom. List your wants and worries, hopes and dreams, about what has been and what you want for your baby, and for the forever changed new YOU.

Words from the YOU after...BABY

_____
_____
_____
_____
_____
_____
_____
_____
_____
_____
_____
_____
_____
_____
_____
_____
_____
_____

About the Author

ON a mission to create books to guide women through major life transitions with insight and humour, Sally founded The YOU After. This is her second book of the series; her first journal The YOU After...WE was the inspiration for *her* new life transition: to publish what seems to be supportive and sassy wisdom, a few sketch emojis, and some blank lines?!

After her idealistic, planned, and stable life became derailed, Sally thought she needed to try something different. She decided to take the opportunity to follow her passion of sharing unsolicited thoughts to, well, anyone who will listen. That's right— it dawned on her that you can block texts, but you can't block freedom of speech in a published book.

Her inspiration to smile, laugh, and gab comes naturally from her family and what she is still trying to prove, some ancestry with clown roots.

But most of all she is driven by the unconditional love for her two beautiful daughters and darling dog (not necessarily in that order ;) She happily resides in her home in Toronto, Canada, with maybe, just maybe, one more home renovation project on the horizon.

For more unsolicited words of questionable wisdom and "dog walking" generated thoughts, please visit her website:

TheYouAfter.com

www.ingramcontent.com/pod-product-compliance
Lightning Source LLC
Chambersburg PA
CBHW020907080526
44589CB00011B/475